How to live a healthy life

6 Simple Ways to Improve Your Health

Arthur Tovar

BSc, D.C. Hons, CSCP, Craniopath Chiropractor

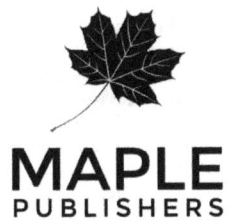

MAPLE
PUBLISHERS

How to live a healthy life

Author: Arthur Tovar

Copyright © 2025 Arthur Tovar

First Published in 2025

ISBN 978-1-83538-778-8 (Paperback)

Cover Design and Book Layout by:
   Maple Publishers
   www.maplepublishers.com

Book Cover Design and Layout by:
   Maple Publishers
   www.maplepublishers.com

Published by:
   Maple Publishers
   Fairbourne Drive, Atterbury,
   Milton Keynes,
   MK10 9RG, UK
   www.maplepublishers.com

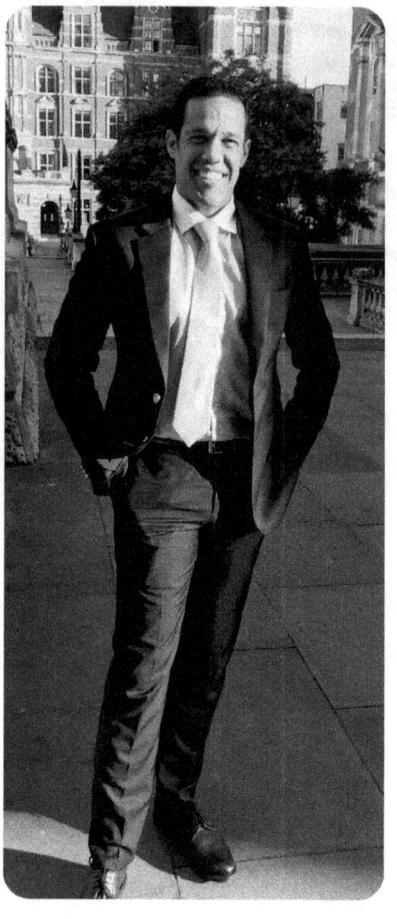

The views expressed in this work are solely those of the author and do not reflect the opinions of Publishers, and the Publisher hereby disclaims any responsibility for them. This book should not be used as a substitute for the advice of a competent authority, admitted or authorized to advise on the subjects covered.
The right of Arthur Tovar to be identified as author of this work has been asserted by the author in accordance with section 77 and 78 of the Copyright, Designs and Patents Act 1988.
The author and publisher have provided this book to you exclusively for your personal use. You may not make this book available to the public in any way. Copyright infringement is punishable by law. If you believe the copy of this book you are reading infringes the author's rights, please notify the publisher.

Dedication

Dedicated to my readers; may this information be valuable and beneficial to your health and well-being.

Recognitions

Thanks to my beautiful wife for without her support and patience this book would not have been possible.

Thanks to my sister Aura Tovar who inspired me to go into Chiropractic School. I borrowed from her strength and inspiration in being an amazing Chiropractor in Miami, Fl.

Thanks to the rest of my family and loved ones for always being there for me and supporting me, both in the best times and the toughest.

Thanks my best Friend Simon Marmier for given me the strength and tenacity to push me through Chiropractic School and beyond. He has inspired me to always be better and reach beyond.

Thanks my mentors, Dr Jonathan Howat, Dr Stephen Williams, Dr Martin Rosen and all my teachers in Chiropractic school. Their teachings have shape the Chiropractor I am today and continues to touch the lives of all the people I have been able to help throughout the years.

Thank you to all the people who have trusted and continue to trust me with their health and the health of their families.

Thanks to my team that without their help and support I would not been able to reach so many in need of Chiropractic care.

Thanks to Pam at Maple Publishing for being patient with me and for making sense of my writing into proper English. Plus everyone involved in the creation of this book, from writing to editing, printing, and publishing.

Arthur Tovar online

Want to send me a WhatsApp message, visit my website, watch my YouTube channel, or follow me on Facebook? Simply scan the QR code with your phone and you'll have access to all platforms.

You can also find more information at www.thamechiropracticclinic.com

Contents

Prologue 7

The disease of modern medicine 8

The crisis of medicine for the sick 11

Health care/Patient care 18

Chiropractic and health 21

Exercise – The energiser of life 28

The change of attitude – The empowerment of life 40

Living Foods – The Essence of Life 47

Time - The enigma of life 62

Water – The elixir of life 68

Farewell words 73

About the Author 75

Prologue

The human body is the most incredible piece of machinery ever created; so complex that no supercomputer can match it.

Billions of cells work in harmony, giving you life and health thanks to an incredibly advanced neurological network that controls all their functions.

But even though it's delivered to us in perfect working order, too often we take it for granted, use it, and abuse it until it breaks down, and only then do we try to find a solution.

Health and well-being don't come from being reactive and trying to fix what's broken, but from being proactive and discovering what benefits us and adding more of it to our lives.

It seems simple:

—Do what is good and beneficial for your body, it will work and you will be fine.

—Do what is bad and harmful to your body and you will suffer, feel sick, and be ill.

As simple as it may be, it is not an easy task.

After being a chiropractor for so many years and seeing thousands of patients, I can tell you that I sincerely wish this body of ours came with a manual so we would all know how to use it properly and, more importantly, take care of it so it stays good for as long as possible.

This book is the manual you should have received when you were born. Better late than never!

Are you ready to discover how you can dramatically improve your health and well-being?

The disease of modern medicine

"I think the biggest problem with medicine today isn't its cost—which is a big problem—but that for all that money, it doesn't express our humanity."
~Jonathan Bush.

"The government doesn't solve problems, it subsidises them."
~Ronald Reagan.

The most significant problems facing the healthcare system worldwide are the same: high costs, poor outcomes, frequent medical errors, and patient dissatisfaction. [1]At the same time, we are facing a global epidemic of obesity and chronic diseases. For example, cardiovascular and respiratory diseases, cancer, dementia, and mental disorders were the leading causes of death in the UK between 2001 and 2018.[2]

The structure and function of the modern healthcare system was established in the early 20th century. Greater emphasis was placed on an acute care approach and much less on prevention and public health. The primary emphasis was on understanding and treating infectious diseases, as well as supporting laboratory research.[3]

---

[1] Fuster V, Kelly BB, editors. *Promoting Cardiovascular Health in the Developing World: a critical challenge to achieve global health*. Washington, DC: The National Academies Press, Institute of Medicine; 2010. https://www.ncbi.nlm.nih.gov/books/NBK45693/

[2] https://www.ons.gov.uk/people population and community/health and social care / causes of death /articles /leading causes of death uk /2001 to 2018

[3] Fleming D, William H. *Welch and the rise of modern medicine*. Boston, Massachusetts: Little, Brown; 1954.

This strategy made sense 100 years ago, given the prevalence of acute infectious diseases in a young population. However, it no longer makes sense. With the aging of the population, the burden of disease has shifted toward chronic conditions. The most common causes of death now are obesity and cigarette smoking, both of which result in delayed but progressive disease. [4]Even in the developing world, chronic diseases are slowly overtaking acute infectious diseases.[5]

The main characteristic of modern medicine is that it uses a dislocated, task-based system aimed at treating acute conditions. It only comes into action after an asymptomatic person becomes ill and requires medication. This system favours specialties over general medicine and procedures over cognitive tasks—that is, surgery over guidance for behaviour modification.

Additionally, the modern medical system relies on new and expensive technology, even though its benefits are not clearly understood. Many low-cost preventive strategies are not researched or adopted because they cannot be patented or converted into revenue.

For example, between 2014 and 2020, total healthcare spending in the UK has grown exponentially. This period has seen restrictions on the growth of National Insurance payments, staff cuts, and a marked increase in waiting times. As a result, funding has increasingly focused on day-to-day expenses to the detriment of broader investment in National Insurance.

Modern medical research typically focuses on solving isolated, short-term problems with 'panacea' solutions. Often, the model for treating an acute infectious disease is applied to treating chronic diseases. For example, chemotherapy for cancer is modelled after antibiotic therapy, and coronary artery bypass grafting mimics the incision and debridement procedure.

---

4   Mokdad AH, Marks JS, Stroup DF, Gerberding JL. *Actual causes of death in the United States*, 2000. JAMA. 2004;291:1238–45. https://www.ncbi.nlm.nih.gov/pubmed/15010446
5   https://www.ncbi.nlm.nih.gov/books/NBK45693/

Changing this broken healthcare system requires changes in medical education, medical research, health policies, and insurance. The current fragmentation of healthcare should be replaced with a patient-centred approach that addresses the whole person. For example, the government should support research into the development and dissemination of prevention strategies and reward the use of appropriate, non-patentable therapies. Primary care physicians should act as health *coaches*, and all medical professionals should adopt a coordinated, multidisciplinary team approach.

Medical education should include preventive strategies, such as lifestyle modification. Rather than limiting itself to diagnosing and managing diseases, it should emphasise homeostasis, wellness, and the practice of low-cost health promotion.

Although the need to manage acute conditions will remain, promoting positive health is the only way to halt the emerging pandemic of chronic disease.

The crisis of medicine for the sick

"If our goal is to destroy the world—to cause global warming, toxicity, and endocrine disruption—we're doing very well."
~William McDonough.

"I want to talk to you about one of the biggest myths in medicine, and that's the idea that we just need more medical discoveries and all our problems will be solved."
~Quien Nguyen.

Our current healthcare system focuses not on maintaining health, but on treating disease, which relies on expensive medications and invasive surgeries. The mission of the current healthcare system seems to be maximising profits rather than helping people maintain or regain their health.

Not only is our healthcare system mediocre to poor, but many of us don't have easy access to it.

Hospitals are also failing to meet several targets, including waiting times for cancer treatment and non-urgent surgeries, such as cataract removal, hernia repairs, and hip and knee replacements, which also takes too long.

The most important points are:
1. **Fewer people are receiving health care.**
   This is due to the high cost of modern medicine.

2. **Lack of regular, scheduled access to a primary health care provider.**

Doctors often do not know important information about their patients' medical history, which affects the quality of medical care.

3. **Difficult access to health care.**

For example, a very small percentage of patients can see a doctor the same day they need it. Access to medical care outside of office hours (early morning, late evening, or on weekends and holidays) is even more difficult. And when a patient needs to go to an emergency room, they often have to wait hours.

4. **Poor management of health care.**

Communication gaps, redundant medical examinations, difficult access to medical records, and breach of confidentiality.

5. **Medical errors.**

These include hospital-acquired infections, adverse reactions to medications, inappropriate medical treatments, unnecessary surgeries, and operations on the wrong parts of the body.

6. **Doctors don't listen to their patients.**

Patient satisfaction is also related to how well their doctors explain things to them, how much time they spend with them, and how they handle their appointments.

7. **High rates of chronic diseases.**

This indicates a lack of attention to lifestyle habits such as diet, exercise, sleep, and stress management.

8. **Most people are dissatisfied with the current health system.**

Especially in the UK where a broken National Health System can barely handle the load of patients that need care.

9. **Giving a Diagnosis/Label is not the only means to a solution.**

The Healthcare system believes that they have done their job once they identify the name/label of a problem. While this usually is half of the solution, it is not the end of the solution.

Usually this leads the patient to bounce to another practitioner that will confirm the diagnoses or label and be given drugs, surgery or another invasive treatment instead of looking at the body as a whole and ask why this happened to begin with?

Is a Headache a Lack of Pain meds? Is an inflammation in the body a lack of steroids or rather a lack of your body's ability to produce natural antiinflammatories called prostaglandins?

For example why do I have Diverticulitis, Pancreatitis, an Ulcer, arthritis in my joints, an Iron deficiency, malaise, etc. What is causing these symptoms and how did they begin?

Few dare to ask why I have XYZ disease and how it began and why it manifested in my body. How can I address those questions? rather than trying to eliminate the symptoms of the disease.

Some of the biggest problems facing our healthcare system are:

1. Chronic illness

For example, in the United Kingdom, one of the biggest health problems is **obesity**. The statistics are alarming.

- In 2017, **64%** of adults in the UK were overweight or obese.
- Overall, **67% of men and 62% of women** are classified as overweight or obese.
- 20% of 6-year-old children are classified as obese.
- **711,000** hospital admissions where obesity was reported as a contributing factor, an increase of 15% from 2016 to 2017.
- **10,660** hospital admissions directly related to obesity in 2017/18, just 100 fewer than in 2016.
- Twenty-**nine percent** of adults are obese, an increase from 26 percent in 2016.[6]

Unfortunately, the obesity epidemic has led to an even more dangerous disorder: **metabolic syndrome**. The World Health Organisation and other

---

6 https://www.finder.com/uk/health-statistics

medical groups, especially the ATP-III, published the concept of metabolic syndrome in 2002 to diagnose and treat increased cardiometabolic risk (previously known as **Syndrome X**).

Metabolic syndrome consists of one of these five variables:
- Obesity.
- Hyperglycaemia (high blood sugar).
- Hypertension (high blood pressure).
- Hypertriglyceridemia (high levels of fat in the blood).
- Low HDL [7](low levels of good cholesterol).

According to the National Cholesterol Education Programme's ATP III guidelines on high blood cholesterol, a person has metabolic syndrome if three of the following conditions are present:

Risk factor	Defining level
Abdominal obesity*	(waist circumference)
Men	>102 cm
Women	>88 cm
Fasting glucose	>110 mg/dL
Blood pressure	>130/>85 mmHg
Triglycerides	>150 mg/dL
HDL cholesterol-	(mg/dL)
Men	<40 mg/dL
Women	<50 mg/dL

Risk factors for metabolic syndrome (minimum three)

*Overweight and obesity are associated with insulin resistance and metabolic syndrome. However, the presence of abdominal obesity is more closely related to metabolic risk factors than a high body mass index (BMI).

---

[7] https://www.ncbi.nlm.nih.gov/pubmed/17469345

Therefore, simple waist circumference measurement is recommended to identify the weight component of metabolic syndrome.

Metabolic syndrome is becoming increasingly common; its presence, or the presence of any of its components, indicates an increased risk of developing complications such as type 2 diabetes and heart disease. However, positive lifestyle changes can delay or even reverse the development of serious health problems.

Another serious medical problem in the world is **cancer**. Cancer is the second leading cause of death in the world, just behind heart disease. [8]The number of new cancer diagnoses in the world is constantly increasing. This rise in cancer incidence is an indication of a sick society living in an unhealthy environment.

2. The opioid crisis

Opioids are a group of pain-relieving medications found naturally in the opium poppy plant. They can be manufactured from the opium poppy plant (morphine) or synthesised in a laboratory (fentanyl). Opioids are used to relieve acute pain and end-of-life pain, but there is little evidence that they are useful for long-term pain relief.[9]

In fact, doctors who specialise in pain management have said that there is no evidence of their effectiveness, but there is potential for harm when prescribing opioids for long-term pain relief.[10] Despite this, opioids are commonly prescribed for long-term pain relief.

This clearly shows that our healthcare system is focusing on the symptom, rather than the problem. Pain is nothing more than a symptom that tells us something is wrong. Pain is not the problem. Instead, we need to address the real problem.

---

8   https://www.bbc.co.uk/news/health-47371078
9   https://www.rcoa.ac.uk/faculty-of-pain-medicine/opioids-aware
10 https://www.bmj.com/content/352/bmj.i20

3. Mental disorders

Depression is considered the second leading cause of disability worldwide and a major contributor to suicide and ischemia. For example, in the United Kingdom, mental health is as follows:

- **1 in 6** people experienced a common mental health problem in the past week.
- It is reported that **1 in 5 women** has mental health problems.
- It is reported that **1 in 8 men** has mental health problems.
- **5,821 suicides** were reported in the UK in 2017.
- **75%** of these suicides in the UK were men.[11]

Additionally, dementia and Alzheimer's disease were the leading causes of death in the UK in 2017 (12.7% of total deaths).

4. Decreased quality of life

Some data show that **life expectancy** could be reduced by problems such as obesity, diabetes, dementia, and, in general, poor lifestyle habits.

Stress: A survey of 2,000 people in Great Britain revealed that 37% of British residents feel stressed at least one full day per week. Women were significantly more prone to stress than men: they suffered from stress three more days per month than men. The most common cause of stress is money, followed by work, health worries, not getting enough sleep, and the pressure of household chores.[12] We can extrapolate from this data and intuit that the figures are very similar in Spain.

The **Mental Health Foundation** commissioned another stress survey between March 29 and April 20, 2018. A total of 4,619 adults were surveyed online. The results are representative of all adults (aged 18 and over) and the results were as follows:

- 74% of adults felt so stressed at some point in the past year that they felt overwhelmed or unable to cope.

---

[11] https://www.finder.com/uk/health-statistics
[12] https://www.forthwithlife.co.uk/blog/great-britain-and-stress/

- 32% of adults said they had experienced suicidal feelings as a result of stress.
- 16% of adults said they had harmed themselves as a result of stress.

Following the survey, Isabella Goldie, director of the Mental Health Foundation, said:

Millions of us are experiencing high levels of stress, and it's damaging our health. Stress is one of the great public health challenges of our time, but it's still not being taken as seriously as concern about physical health.

Stress is a significant factor in mental health problems, including anxiety and depression. It's also linked to physical health issues, such as heart disease, problems with our immune system, insomnia, and digestive problems. Individually, we need to understand what's causing us stress and learn what steps we can take to reduce it in ourselves and those around us.[13]

Burnout: The World Health Organisation has now officially recognised burnout as an occupational phenomenon, describing it as a "syndrome resulting from occupational stress that has not been successfully managed." It is characterised by:

- Feeling exhausted.
- Negativism or cynicism about work.
- Poor work performance.

Causes of burnout include unreasonable pressure, unmanageable workload, lack of support from managers, and a toxic work culture.

Although there are no statistics available on the prevalence of burnout specifically, it is estimated that 45% of employees in Spain suffer from work-related stress.[14]

---

13 https://www.mentalhealth.org.uk/publications/stress-are-we-coping
14 https://www.observatoriorh.com/orh-posts/45-per-cent-of-workers-suffer-work-stress.html

Health care/Patient care

"We are not tinsmiths who simply patch and heal what is broken... we must be vigilant, guardians of the life and health of our generation, so that stronger and more capable generations may come after us."

~Dr. Elizabeth Blackwell (1821–1910), Anglo-American physician and the first female medical doctor in modern times.

"The enjoyment of the highest attainable standard of health is one of the fundamental rights of every human being, regardless of race, religion, political beliefs, or economic or social conditions."

~World Health Organisation.

Who is responsible for the state of our healthcare system? As Walter Cronkite ironically said, "The United States healthcare system is neither healthy, nor caring, nor a system." That's why conventional medicine is now called sick care.

We tend to blame it on:
- **The Government**, for the poor management of Social Security.
- **The pharmaceutical industry**, for its cynical marketing practices to doctors.
- **The food industry**, for the production of highly processed and unhealthy food.
- **The patient care system**, due to its emphasis on crisis management rather than the promotion of positive health practices.

The goal of the patient care system is to take the patient from **-7 (fighting) to 0 (surviving)**. Its ideal is a 'pain-free' state.

For example, if you have a disorder that affects your health, the healthcare system will prescribe a medication that will relieve or reduce your symptoms. However, that medication likely won't eliminate the underlying cause of your disorder. Therefore, you may need to continue taking that medication as long as the disorder persists, and you'll also have to deal with the side effects it causes. And even if you have a slightly better quality of life, you'll still have to rely on medication to get through each day.

On the other hand, the goal of true healthcare is to transform each patient from **0 (survival) to +7 (well-being)**. Your ideal is 'well-being': maximised performance and optimised potential.

This ideal is aligned with the World Health Organisation's definition of health: **'Health is a state of complete physical, mental and social well-being and not merely the absence of disease or infirmity'.** [15]

This ideal of health benefits most from personalised medicine because it offers a combination of conventional medical therapies and complementary therapies supported by high-quality scientific evidence of their safety and effectiveness. Personalised medicine is oriented toward healing, taking into account the whole person, including all aspects of lifestyle. It emphasises the therapeutic relationship between practitioner and patient, is informed by evidence, and utilises all appropriate therapies.[16]

I believe in personalised healthcare so you can achieve the highest levels of health. Our consultation goals are:

- Discover the underlying cause of the health problem.
- Suggest a care plan that will produce the best results.
- Provide ways for patients to participate in their own recovery.
- Explain the value of post-symptomatic wellness care.

---

[15] Preamble to the WHO Constitution, adopted by the International Health Conference, New York, 19 June–22 July 1946; signed on 22 July 1946 by the representatives of 61 States (Official Records of WHO, No. 2, p. 100) and entered into force on 7 April 1948. The definition has not been amended since 1948.

[16] The University of Arizona Center of Integrative Medicine. *What is Integrative Medicine?* https://integrativemedicine.arizona.edu/about/definition.html

We help you shift from a healthcare model predominantly based on disease management (waiting for symptoms and then taking action) to a tailored wellness model that suits you.

In this book, we'll explain the vital principles that will help you achieve your health goals. These are:
— Chiropractic and health.
— Exercise.
— The change in attitude.
— Food.
— The weather.
— Hydration.

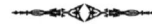

Chiropractic and health

"If there is a definition of healing, it is to touch with compassion and awareness those pains that we have turned away from with prejudice and dismay."
~Stephen Levine.
"Preserving health is easier than curing disease."
~Bartlett Joshua Palmer.

Chiropractic

"I've been visiting chiropractors forever. It's as important to my training as practising my *swing*."
~Tiger Woods.
"Study the spine to know the cause of the disease."
~Hippocrates.

The word **chiropractic** comes from the Greek and means 'done by hand'. The practice originated in 1895 with Daniel David Palmer, a self-taught healer from Iowa. He was searching for a cure for ailments and diseases that wasn't based on drugs or surgery. Palmer invented chiropractic by curing the deafness of a man who had lost his hearing after over exerting himself with heavy labour. Palmer attributed the hearing loss to a displaced vertebra and corrected it by adjusting the man's spine.

Based on this and other cases he treated with spinal adjustments, Palmer proposed his theory that most diseases are caused by misaligned vertebrae affecting the nerves of the spine. These misalignments are called subluxations. Correcting these misalignments restores normal nerve and brain function and allows the body to heal.

Through advances in research and a greater understanding of how the body works, we have learned that when the spine is misaligned and not moving properly (the causes of which can be physical, chemical, or emotional), the brain receives a distorted image of what the body is doing and how it is functioning. This results in a state of poor communication, misinterpretation, and maladaptation, leaving the body in a state of stress and dysfunction. It has been proven that through specific, targeted, and repeated spinal adjustments, the brain and body become more 'connected', resulting in an optimised state of function and maximum potential. This greatly improves quality of life and contributes to reducing the symptoms that many patients experience.

Chiropractors adjust the spine using their hands, applying force and pressure to areas that are out of alignment or do not have a normal range of motion.

After physicians and dentists, chiropractors are the third largest group of healthcare providers who directly care for patients. The American Medical Association (AMA) policy currently establishes that it is ethical for physicians not only to associate professionally with chiropractors but also to refer their patients to them for diagnostic or therapeutic services.

Family physicians are the physicians most likely to refer patients to chiropractors, followed by family nurse practitioners, internists, neurologists, neurosurgeons, gynaecologists, and general surgeons. Chiropractors also frequently refer their patients to other health care providers.[17]

Chiropractors see patients with problems such as:
- Back pain/lumbago.
- Neck pain/cervicalgia.
- Joint pain (shoulders, elbows, wrists, hips, knees, ankles).
- Headaches/migraines.

---

[17] Christensen MG, Kollasch MW, Hyland JK. «Practice analysis of chiropractic», 2010. *A project report, survey analysis, and summary of the practice of chiropractic within the United States*. Greeley, CO: National Board of Chiropractic Examiners; 2010

- Dizziness/vertigo.
- Sciatica.
- Disc protrusion/herniation.
- General pain.
- Stress.

Since chiropractic adjustments focus on reducing neurological interference at the level of the spine and since the nervous system controls the entire body, many people report noticing positive changes and improvements in their body's functioning, such as at the following levels:

- Respiratory.
- Cardiovascular.
- Digestive.
- Urinary function.
- Sexual function.
- Dream.
- Energy.
- Immune function.

Chiropractors also treat children from birth to counteract the impact that the stress of childbirth can have on their spines and to support them throughout their growth to ensure they do not develop spinal problems.

Chiropractic is proven to be safe and effective for the health and well-being of human beings from newborns to the elderly.

In Spain, the profession is growing rapidly, with more and more people seeking chiropractic care not only to reduce pain or stress, but also to maximise their potential and enjoy a better quality of life.

Vitalism

The term vitalism means belief in the body's innate ability to heal itself. It recognises and respects the intelligent order of the universe and the body (as opposed to a state of disorganised chaos). It acknowledges that life is fully expressed through order and harmony. Vitalism understands that interference with this order will result in a state of malaise.

According to Life University, "Our bodies work hard to express health, to maintain health, and to recover from illness or other conditions that threaten our health." For chiropractors who follow the vitalistic paradigm of thinking, the primary goal of an adjustment is to allow for the restoration of order, so that the intelligent brain sees the body correctly and, therefore, allows healing to occur naturally, as it should.

It's easier to believe in vitalism when you're young. Your body feels youthful and resilient. In this state of mind, you don't doubt your body's ability to return to a healthy state. You simply let your body do its thing, without interference.

As an alternative philosophical viewpoint, mechanism views the body as a series of mechanical systems, such as the pulmonary or cardiovascular systems, and treats them as separate entities. Mechanism is best understood as referring to allopathic medicine, where symptoms are addressed as the primary focus, and once symptoms have been reduced and managed, further intervention or treatment is discontinued.

There are elements of truth in both vitalism and mechanism. You can honour the body's ability to participate in its own healing. At the same time, you can respect what mechanists do and look for ways to work with those ideas, rather than against them. Let common sense and facts guide you toward a rational decision. Emphasise evidence-based and patient-centred medicine. Focus on what works and is supported by clinical evidence. Indeed, optimal care should be based on the best available evidence and the best outcomes.[18]

Personally, I have a vitalist approach to health. I respect and understand the role of the mechanistic perspective and work with all healthcare colleagues. My goal is simply to bring my patients to a healthy state.

---

[18] https://www.chiroeco.com/vitalism-vs-mechanism-a-fresh-view/

Health in the community

"The power of the community to create health is far greater than that of any single doctor, clinic, or hospital."

~Dr. Mark Hyman.

"The need for connection and community is paramount, as fundamental as the need for air, water, and food."

~Dr. Dean Ornish.

A healthy community is one in which groups from all walks of life work together to prevent disease and establish healthy lifestyle choices. Community-based health care provides the greatest possible benefits to as many people as possible. It also helps reduce health gaps caused by differences in income, education, race and ethnicity, location, and other factors.

To improve the health of your community, start by taking care of yours and your family's. Make sure you're as healthy as possible with the help of proper nutrition, daily physical activity, and regular chiropractic checkups.

Then, help promote health in your community by becoming more involved. Encourage local community groups and government organisations to consider community health in their plans.[19]

Promoting and maintaining a healthy community concerns everyone and is the responsibility of every individual who lives within it. In the words of Coretta Scott King: "The greatness of a community is most accurately measured by the compassionate actions of its members."

Health in the family

"Medicine cannot work without family."

~Carol Levine

The importance of family in well-being

In health, the importance of family is evident. Family support can provide comfort, support, and even influence better health outcomes

---

[19] https://blogs.cdc.gov/publichealthmatters/2015/09/a-healthy-community-is-a-prepared-community/

when you're not feeling well. Families establish patterns of preventive care, exercise, hygiene, and responsibility. They also lay the foundation for self-esteem, resilience, and the ability to form healthy, empathetic relationships.[20]

All the healthiest and longest-lived people in the world have one thing in common: they put their families first. One of the biggest challenges families face in staying connected is the hectic pace of life. Author Mimi Doe recommends connecting with your family by spending time together and expressing love and support for one another. It's also important to let go of petty grievances.[21]

The same practices apply to relationships with close friends. This is especially important if you don't have any living family or live far away from them.

Love and health

"The best and most beautiful things in the world are not seen, nor even heard, but are felt with the heart."

~Helen Keller.

"There are too many people looking for the perfect person, instead of trying to be the right person."

~Gloria Steinem.

According to a growing body of scientific research, love provides exceptional health benefits. Dr. Helen Riess, director of the Empathy and Relational Science Program at Massachusetts General Hospital, lists these five health benefits of love:

1. Love makes you happy.

---

[20] https://www.takingcharge.csh.umn.edu/create-healthy-lifestyle/relationships/why-relationships-family-are-important/-importance-family-wel

[21] https://www.takingcharge.csh.umn.edu/nurture-your-relationships

In the first moments of falling in love, dopamine is activated, the happy chemical in the brain associated with reward. It makes us feel positive and appreciated, and this, naturally, is good for our health.

2. Love repels stress.

After the initial phase, another brain chemical, oxytocin or the bonding hormone, is activated. This reduces stress levels and creates greater homeostasis and balance.

3. Love relieves anxiety.

Being in love and feeling close to another person can reduce the anxiety caused by loneliness and insecurity.

4. Love makes us take better care of ourselves.

Couples encourage each other to go to the doctor when they don't want to. Sometimes, partners even notice early signs of a health problem before the person with the problem does.

5. Love helps you live longer.

Research has shown that married couples enjoy greater longevity than single couples due to consistent social and emotional support and better adherence to medical care. [22]Likewise, a partner will hold you accountable for leading a healthy lifestyle and steer you away from destructive behaviours . Married couples have a lower incidence of substance abuse, [23]as well as lower blood pressure and less depression [24]than unmarried couples.[25]

In the words of Sophocles: "One word frees us from all the weight and pain of life. That word is love."

---

22 https://time.com/3706692/do-married-people-really-live-longer/
23 https://www.ncbi.nlm.nih.gov/pmc/articles/PMC1449833/
24 https://academic.oup.com/abm/article/35/2/239/4569261
25 https://time.com/5136409/health-benefits-love/

Exercise – The energiser of life

"Your body will get better at whatever you do, or don't do. Not moving? Your body will get better at the art of NOT moving. If you move, your body will allow you more movement."

~ Ido Portal.

"For wild animals, movement isn't a chore, it's not a temporary punishment for being physically lazy and out of shape, it's not an optional activity just to look better."

~ Erwan Le Corre.

Modern man movement / Pre-industrial man movement

Before the Industrial Revolution, strenuous physical activity was a normal part of our ancestors' daily lives. They worked hard to feed themselves and provide shelter and security for the community. But their physical exertion was not limited to the demands of their working lives. In those days, people engaged in one- or two-day periods of intense and strenuous effort, followed by one- or two-day periods of rest and celebration.

However, even during these so-called days of rest, they would make visiting trips of 10 to 40 kilometres to see relatives or friends and to trade with other clans or communities. They also participated in dances and other social activities.[26]

---

[26] U.S. Department of Health and Human Services. *Physical Activity and Health: A Report of the Surgeon General.* Atlanta, GA: U.S. Department of Health and Human Services, Centers for Disease Control and Prevention, National Center for Chronic Disease Prevention and Health Promotion, 1996

Today, our physical activity is much lower than that of our pre-industrial ancestors. Thanks to modern technology, we have low levels of physical activity and high levels of sedentary behaviour. According to WHO estimates, approximately one in five adults globally was not sufficiently active in 2010 (20% of men and 27% of women).[27]

"In less than two generations, physical activity has declined by 20% in the United Kingdom and 32% in the United States. In China, the decline is 45% in less than a generation. Vehicles, machines, and technology now move for us. What we do in our free time doesn't come close to making up for what we've lost."[28]

The biggest obstacle preventing us from walking or doing other types of physical activity is lack of time. Regular aerobic physical activity has to compete with the demands of home, work, school, and the community.

We are still designed to move, not to stay still.

"The truth about the human species is that in body, spirit, and behaviour, we are designed to grow and develop in ways that emphasise, rather than minimise, childlike traits. We are supposed to remain childlike in many ways; we were never meant to 'grow up' and become the kind of adults most of us are today."

~Ashley Montagu.

The human body functions best when it's active. From an evolutionary perspective, we're designed to move: to move around and engage in all kinds of manual labor throughout the day. This was essential for our survival as a species. The recent shift from a physically demanding life to a sedentary one has been relatively sudden.

Furthermore, over the past 20 years, the amount of time we've spent in front of screens (smartphones, computers, televisions, and video games) and driving has increased dramatically. The health consequences of a sedentary lifestyle cannot be reversed with exercise. Therefore, we must reduce the total amount of time we spend sitting, in addition to engaging

---

[27] https://www.who.int/news-room/fact-sheets/detail/physical-activity
[28] https://www.icsspe.org/bookshop/designed-move

in moderate to vigorous exercise. Parents often tell their children to go outside and play. Adults need similar advice from their doctors![29]

Sitting or standing

"Sitting is the new smoking."

~Dr. James Levine.

Excessive sitting has been linked to an increased risk of early death. [30]Sitting for long periods leads to tightness of the abdominal and hamstring muscles and affects the lower back. Using a standing desk for a while can help maintain better spinal alignment and muscle symmetry. However, standing all day isn't ideal either. Taking frequent breaks is the best way to ensure you're sitting or standing optimally. Also, pay attention to your posture: the top of your computer screen should be roughly at eye level.

Interrupting sitting with periods of standing or short walks relieves pain and fatigue, and improves control of blood sugar, blood pressure, and weight gain.

Watching TV or playing games while standing is also a good way to reduce the amount of time we spend sitting. However, the potential benefits of standing instead of sitting need further study.[31]

Types of exercise and their benefits

"If you only have time to exercise or meditate, but not both, then make exercise your daily meditation."

~ Steve Pavlina

Strengthening, stretching, balance, and aerobic exercises are the four most important types of exercise, which keep you active, mobile, and feeling great.

---

[29] https://www.ncbi.nlm.nih.gov/pmc/articles/PMC2996155/
[30] http://annals.org/aim/article-abstract/2653704/patterns-sedentary-behavior-mortality-u-s-middle-aged-older-adults
[31] https://www.healthline.com/health-news/debate-over-standing

1. Aerobic exercises

Aerobic exercise increases your heart and breathing rates and increases endurance. Aim for 150 minutes of moderate to vigorous activity per week, such as brisk walking, swimming, jogging, cycling, dancing, or classes like *step aerobics*.

2. Strength training

As we age, we lose muscle mass. Strength training restores it. Exercising your muscles not only makes you stronger, but also stimulates bone growth, lowers blood sugar, helps with weight control, improves balance and posture, and reduces stress and pain in the lower back and joints. Strength training includes weight-bearing exercises such as squats, push-ups, and lunges, as well as exercises against resistance from a dumbbell, resistance band, or weight machine.

3. Stretching

Aging brings with it a loss of flexibility in muscles and tendons. Stretching helps improve flexibility, increases your range of motion, and reduces pain and the risk of injury. You need to stretch all parts of your body every day. Start by warming up your muscles, then perform static stretches for up to 60 seconds on your calves, hips, lower back, shoulders, arms, and neck.

4. Balance exercises

Improving your balance helps prevent falls, which is especially important as we age. If you're afraid of falling, consult a professional, who will determine your current balance skills and prescribe specific exercises to target your weak areas. Balance exercises include standing on one foot or walking heel to toe, with your eyes open or closed, and walking on uneven surfaces. Yoga or tai chi classes are also good options for improving balance.[32]

---

[32] https://www.health.harvard.edu/exercise-and-fitness/the-4-most-important-types-of-exercise

Most people tend to focus on one activity or type of exercise and think they're doing enough. However, every type of exercise is different. Doing a little bit of everything will give you greater benefits. Mixing things up also helps reduce boredom and your risk of injury. Additionally, some activities fit into more than one category. For example, many resistance activities also build strength. And some strengthening exercises can also help improve balance and flexibility.[33]

1. Yoga

Yoga is a mind-body practice that combines physical postures, breathing exercises, and relaxation. Yoga develops flexibility, endurance, balance, and muscular strength. Yoga practice has been shown to increase awareness not only in class but also in other areas of a person's life. Yoga is now included in many cardiac rehabilitation programmes due to its heart-healthy and stress-relieving benefits.

There are many types of yoga. Hatha yoga (a combination of many styles) is one of the most popular. Hatha yoga focuses on *pranayama* (breath-controlled exercises), *asanas* (yoga postures), and *savasanas* (rest periods).[34]

2. Pilates

Pilates is named after its creator, Joseph Pilates, who developed the exercises in the 1920s. Pilates is an exercise method consisting of low-impact flexibility and muscle-strengthening movements, as well as resistance exercises. Pilates emphasises proper postural alignment, core strength, and muscular balance. Many Pilates exercises can be performed on the floor using just a mat.

The health benefits of Pilates include:
- More core strength and stability.
- Improving posture and balance.

---

[33] https://go4life.nia.nih.gov/4-types-of-exercise/
[34] https://www.health.harvard.edu/staying-healthy/yoga-benefits-beyond-the-mat

- Increased flexibility.
- Prevention and treatment of back pain.

However, Pilates does not include aerobic exercise, so you will need to complement it with aerobic exercises, such as brisk walking, jogging, cycling, or swimming.[35]

3. Swimming

Swimming is an excellent exercise because it forces you to move your entire body against the resistance of the water. Swimming is a good all-around activity because:

- Builds endurance, muscle strength and cardiovascular fitness.
- Tones and strengthens muscles.
- Helps maintain body weight, and a healthy heart and lungs.
- It provides a full-body workout, as almost every muscle in the body is used in swimming.[36]

However, the pool can be used not only for swimming, but also for water aerobics, such as walking, jogging, or running underwater, as well as vigorous aerobics. Heated pools can help warm up your joints and muscles. Aquatic exercise can improve physical functioning in adults over 50.[37]

4. Strength training

Strength training should be an important part of every fitness programme. It helps you reduce body fat, increase lean muscle mass, and burn calories more efficiently. Strength training also helps you:

- Develop strong bones.
- Reduce or maintain your weight.

---

[35] https://www.mayoclinic.org/healthy-lifestyle/fitness/in-depth/pilates-for-beginners/art-20047673
[36] https://www.betterhealth.vic.gov.au/health/healthyliving/swimming-health-benefits
[37] https://www.mayoclinic.org/healthy-lifestyle/fitness/in-depth/ready-to-get-in-on-the-aquatic-fitness-movement/art-20390059

- Improve your quality of life.
- Reduce the signs and symptoms of many chronic conditions, including arthritis, back pain, obesity, heart disease, depression, and diabetes.
- Sharpen your thinking and learning skills, and improve your memory.

Strength training can be done at home or at the gym using:
- Bodyweight exercises, such as push-ups, planks, lunges, and squats.
- Free weights, such as barbells and dumbbells.
- Resistance bands, which are lightweight elastic tubes that produce resistance when stretched.
- Exercise machines [38].

5. Crossfit

CrossFit is a training programme that strengthens *and* conditions through extremely varied and demanding workouts.

- Most *CrossFit gyms* separate their classes into three or four sections:
- Dynamic warm-up. This includes jumping jacks, jumping rope, squats, planks, lunges, push-ups, functional movements, stretching, and mobility work.
- Skill or strength work. If it's a strength day, you'll work on pure strength movements, such as squats or deadlifts. If it's not a strength day, you'll work on a skill, such as single-leg squats.
- Workout of the day. You'll either do a certain number of repetitions of a particular exercise as quickly as you can, or you'll have a time limit to do as many repetitions of a particular exercise as possible.
- Cool down and stretch.

---

[38] https://www.mayoclinic.org/healthy-lifestyle/fitness/in-depth/strength-training/art-20046670

A word of caution: *CrossFit* isn't for everyone. If you have a history of injuries or medical conditions, it may not be the best option for you. Most *CrossFit gyms* will allow you to attend a class for free. If you have a gym nearby, try each one before choosing the one that's best for you.[39]

7. Zumba

Zumba is a fitness programme that combines Latin and international music with dance movements. Zumba can be a moderate or vigorous aerobic activity, depending on its intensity. It incorporates interval training (alternating fast and slow rhythms) and resistance training. The class provides a powerful cardio workout and also helps with coordination and agility. Zumba dance moves are easy to follow and learn. It's a full-body workout, adaptable to any fitness level. The music, energetic atmosphere, group experience, and changing routines will get you sweating, but in a fun way.[40]

8. Core muscle exercises

You use your core muscles to perform daily activities, such as tying your shoes and lifting heavy objects. These muscles also affect your balance, posture, and stability.

Your core muscles include your abs, as well as the muscles in your back and around your pelvis. Strengthening these muscles helps stabilise your body, support your spine, and improve your overall fitness. Core exercises for beginners include push-ups, crunches, bicycle crunches, leg lifts, planks, and boat pose.[41]

9. Fine motor control

Fine motor control is the ability to make small, precise movements, such as picking up a very small object with your thumb and index finger. Damage to the brain, nerves, muscles, or joints due to injury, illness, or

---

[39] https://www.nerdfitness.com/blog/a-beginners-guide-to-crossfit/
[40] https://www.mayoclinic.org/healthy-lifestyle/fitness/expert-answers/zumba/faq-20057883
[41] https://www.stylecraze.com/articles/core-strengthening-exercises

stroke can affect this control. Congenital deformities, cerebral palsy, or developmental disabilities can also be detrimental.

Therapeutic exercises can help improve impaired fine motor control functions. For example, the Stroke Association recommends the following exercises:

- **Forced use:** the Constraint-induced movement therapy is an effective exercise for loss of fine motor control. For example, if you've lost the use of your right hand, you may be able to revert to using your left hand. During constraint-induced movement therapy, your left hand is tied to your side, forcing you to rely on your affected limb for all fine motor tasks. This exercise can be performed for up to six hours a day.
- **Cadences:** Choose a task like inserting pegs into holes. Set a timer and fill all the holes. Repeat this exercise every day, aiming for faster times each day, until you reach your optimal skill level.[42]

When should you exercise?

The best time to exercise is different for everyone. Train at the time that works best for you. The key is to do what's most likely to work for you, because consistency is more important than timing.

For example, you may have heard that the best time to exercise is early in the morning. But if you're not a morning person, you'll find it difficult to get up early to work out. Similarly, if you find that working out late makes you less able to fall asleep, you may need to exercise earlier in the day or try less intense exercises. Finally, if your schedule isn't predictable, or you're travelling, you may need to be flexible and exercise when you can.

There's no perfect time of day to exercise, so do it whenever works best for you.[43]

---

[42] https://www.sportsrec.com/126568-occupational-therapy-exercises-fine-motor.html

[43] https://www.heart.org/en/healthy-living/fitness/fitness-basics/when-is-the-best-time-of-day-to-work-out

Is it necessary to change exercises with age?

We tend to underestimate and undermine the physical potential of older adults. They can definitely exercise, although their flexibility and functional capacity are diminished by age and a sedentary lifestyle. However, it's best to consult a specialist before starting any exercise regimen.

Motivation: Many older adults become anxious, tense, and nervous in an exercise environment, which can make them reluctant to try anything new or different. However, most understand the dangers of inactivity and the benefits of exercise. Their exercise programme should be individualised to help them feel confident and secure. It's important to be encouraging, because older adults often experience self-doubt and uncertainty.

Safety: Safety is the most important concern in exercise programmes for older adults. They should exercise in well-lit areas with easy-to-use equipment. It is important for them to drink water before, during, and after exercise to avoid dehydration. They may also need to wear layered clothing to adjust to varying temperatures. They will need to slow down and stop if they experience any health warning signs during exercise, such as shortness of breath or fatigue.

Set realistic goals: Before starting an exercise programme, it's important to set individualised, realistic, and achievable goals. These goals should begin with low to moderate activity. The overall goal should be to improve strength, flexibility, body composition, and cardiovascular endurance.

Warm-up and flexibility: Each session should begin with a warm-up, such as walking and stretching all joints for 10 or 15 minutes. Similarly, the session should end with a cool-down period, including stretching and relaxation.

Aerobic exercise: Aerobic activities such as walking, swimming, water exercises, and bicycling are appropriate for seniors. Swimming and water exercises place less stress on the joints than stationary biking, while recumbent biking places less stress on the back. Walking at a faster pace than normal can be easily done in most environments and requires no additional equipment.

Strength training: Muscle strength, mobility, and balance can be significantly improved with supervised resistance training. Older adults can perform a resistance exercise programme three times a week. They should be reminded to breathe normally and not hold their breath during resistance exercises.

A sedentary lifestyle leads to instability, premature death, and a poor quality of life. Chronological age does not represent the quality of health, and it is important to note that preventing complications associated with inactivity is much cheaper than the cost of providing long-term care.[44]

The best recommendations

"If there were a pill that contained all the benefits of exercise, this would be the most prescribed medication in the world."

~Dr. Ronald Davis

- Move more and sit less to offset the risk of heart disease, high blood pressure, and mortality due to increased sedentary behavior. Set a timer and take a short walk every 30-45 minutes.
- Move more frequently throughout the day. Integrate movement into your daily life. Take the stairs instead of the elevator. Walk short distances. Exercise while watching TV. Walk while talking on your cell phone.

Optimise your health

To get the best health benefits from physical activity, you need at least 150 to 300 minutes of moderate to vigorous aerobic activity, such as brisk walking or fast dancing, each week. It's also important to do muscle-strengthening exercises, such as planks or weight lifting, at least two days a week.[45]

Both aerobic exercise and strength training are important for improving your endurance and muscle mass. You also need to improve your flexibility and balance. Finding the right balance will depend on your

---

[44] https://www.unm.edu/~lkravitz/Article%20folder/age.html
[45] https://health.gov/paguidelines/second-edition/10things/

individual goals, how quickly you want to achieve them, and the amount of time you can dedicate to the exercises.[46]

Final idea:

"If everyone knew how to use water, half of the ailments due to disease would be eliminated. We would take care of the other half by understanding how and when to eat, how to breathe, and the need for daily exercise." ~Louisa Lust.

---

[46] https://www.healthline.com/health/how-often-should-you-work-out

The change of attitude – The empowerment of life

"The greatest revolution of our generation is the discovery that human beings, by changing the internal attitude of their minds, can change the external aspects of their lives."

~William James.

"A healthy attitude is contagious, but don't wait to catch it from others. Be a carrier."

~ Tom Stoppard .

Mind-body connection

"The brain and peripheral nervous system, the endocrine and immune systems, and indeed all of our body's organs, as well as all of our emotional responses, share a common chemical language and are in constant communication with each other."

~Dr. James Gordon (founder of the Centre for Mind-Body Medicine).

The mind-body connection means that our thoughts, feelings, beliefs, and attitudes can positively or negatively affect the functioning of our bodies. On the other hand, what we eat, how much we exercise, and even our posture can have a positive or negative impact on our mental state. This results in a complex exchange between our minds and our bodies.

Mind-body therapies use the body to influence the mind and vice versa. These include:

- Meditation.
- Prayer.
- Yoga.

- Tai Chi.
- Qigong.
- Biofeedback.
- Relaxation.
- Hypnosis.
- Guided imagery.
- Patient support groups.
- Cognitive behavioural therapy.
- Creative arts therapies (art, music or dance).

Highlight that the mind is not the same as the brain.
- The mind consists of mental states, such as thoughts, emotions, beliefs, attitudes, and images (*software*).
- The brain is the organ that allows us to experience these mental states (*hardware*).

Mental states can be conscious or unconscious. Each mental state has a positive or negative effect on the physical body. For example, the mental state of anxiety causes the production of stress hormones. Many mind-body therapies will help you become more aware of your mental and emotional state. You can use this awareness to guide your thoughts and emotions in a better, more positive direction.[47]

What is a healthy mind?

"The key to a healthy life is a healthy mind."

~Richard Davidson.

A healthy mind is not simply the absence of mental illness. According to the World Health Organisation (WHO), mental health is "a state of well-being in which the individual realises his or her own abilities, can cope with the normal stresses of life, work productively and fruitfully, and is able to contribute to his or her community."[48]

---

[47] https://www.takingcharge.csh.umn.edu/what-is-the-mind-body-connection
[48] World Health Organization. *Promoting mental health: concepts, emerging*

Mental health is a dynamic state of internal stability that allows us to use our abilities in harmony with society's universal values. The components of a healthy mind are:

- A harmonious relationship between body and mind.
- Basic cognitive and social skills.
- The ability to recognise, express and control our own emotions.
- The ability to empathise with the emotions of others.
- The ability to fulfil different social roles.
- The ability and flexibility to deal with adverse life events.[49]

Some steps you can take to develop a healthy mind:
- **Stay active.**
- Movement and exercise lift your spirits. They also help you sleep better and get the rest you need.
- **Reduce your alcohol consumption.**
- Alcohol can increase feelings of depression and also affect your physical health.
- **Connect with family and friends.**
- Spending quality time with your loved ones is the best way to boost your mental well-being.
- **Stay open and curious.**
- Learn a new sport or language, learn to play an instrument, read books, and feed your mind with positive inspiration.[50]

Positive affirmations

Positive affirmations are positive phrases or statements used to reverse negative or unhelpful thoughts. They can be used to reduce stress, boost

---

evidence, practice (Compendium Report). Geneva: World Health Organization; 2004

[49] https://www.ncbi.nlm.nih.gov/pmc/articles/PMC4471980/

[50] https://www.sahealth.sa.gov.au/wps/wcm/connect/Public+Content/SA+Health+Internet/Healthy+living/Healthy+mind/

your self-esteem, or make positive changes in your life. Practising positive affirmations is simple. Choose a positive phrase that resonates with you and repeat it to yourself. However, positive affirmations require regular practice if you want to achieve long-term, sustainable changes.

Positive affirmations are designed to encourage an optimistic mindset. They reduce negative thoughts and the tendency to dwell on negative experiences. When we replace negative messages with positive statements, we can build more hopeful narratives about who we are and what we can achieve.

Positive affirmations are based on the idea that your thoughts can influence your health for the better. You can use them to improve your physical health as well as heal your emotional pain.

For example, here are some of the positive affirmations from author Louise Hay:

1. Life only brings me good experiences. I'm open to new and wonderful changes.
2. I feel a glorious, dynamic energy. I'm active and alive.
3. Each of my experiences is perfect for my growth.
4. Today I create a wonderful day and a wonderful new future.
5. Abundance flows freely in me.
6. My self-esteem is high because I honor the person I am.[51]

Whether you're looking for ways to manage stress or simply want to improve your emotional state, use the affirmations provided or create some of your own.[52]

Pain - the mental component

"Pain is inevitable; suffering is not."

~Buddha.

---

[51] https://www.louisehay.com/affirmations/
[52] https://positivepsychology.com/daily-affirmations/

Pain is defined as "an unpleasant sensory and emotional experience associated with actual or potential tissue damage, or described in terms of such damage." Pain is a bodily sensation and is always an unpleasant emotional experience.

Pain is the primary reason patients seek medical care, and it is one of the most disabling, bothersome, and costly conditions. Pain accompanies many diseases, each of which generates separate diagnostic, therapeutic, and research challenges.[53]

The following factors can affect how we perceive and react to pain:
1. Our beliefs about pain.
2. Our beliefs about our ability to control pain (self-efficacy).
3. Previous experiences with pain.
4. Recovery expectations.
5. Current emotional states, including catastrophising, anxiety, and depression.[54]

Mindfulness. It involves focusing the mind to increase awareness of the present moment. This method can be easily done anywhere to help deal with pain and stress. An example of *mindfulness meditation* would be to sit up straight, close your eyes, and focus your attention on your breathing as you inhale and exhale. This exercise can be done for just a couple of minutes or longer. It helps if you let your thoughts come and go while being aware of your breathing. It can be extremely helpful during times of stress and during difficult life events.

Mindfulness can create a sense of control that helps make your pain experience more manageable. Yoga, tai chi, and other mind-body techniques are also recommended for the same benefits [55].

---

[53] https://www.ncbi.nlm.nih.gov/pubmed/25000837
[54] https://www.physio-pedia.com/Psychological_Basis_of_Pain
[55] https://www.hss.edu/conditions_emotional-impact-pain-experience.asp

Cognitive-behavioural therapy

Cognitive-behavioural therapy (CBT) is a talking therapy that can help you manage your problems by changing the way you think and act. It's most commonly used to treat anxiety and depression. However, it can also be helpful for other physical and mental health issues.

CBT is based on the concept that your thoughts, feelings, physical sensations, and actions are interconnected. CBT aims to help you deal with overwhelming problems in a more positive way by breaking them down into smaller parts. You'll be taught how to change your negative patterns to improve how you feel. CBT addresses your current problems instead of focusing on issues from your past. Look for practical ways to improve your mental state every day.

Uses of CBT

CBT is an effective way to treat a number of different mental health conditions. In addition to depression or anxiety disorders, CBT can also help people with:

- Bipolar disorder.
- Borderline personality disorder.
- Eating disorders, such as anorexia and bulimia.
- Obsessive-compulsive disorder (OCD).
- Panic disorder.
- Phobias.
- Post-traumatic stress disorder (PTSD).
- Problems related to alcohol misuse.
- Psychosis.
- Schizophrenia.
- Sleep problems, such as insomnia.

CBT is sometimes used to treat people with long-term health conditions, such as irritable bowel syndrome (IBS), chronic fatigue syndrome (CFS), and fibromyalgia.

Although CBT cannot cure the physical symptoms of these illnesses, it does help people better cope with their symptoms.

Cognitive behavioural therapy (CBT) can be as effective as medication in treating some mental health problems, but it may not be successful or appropriate for everyone.

Benefits of CBT:
- It can be useful in cases where medicine alone has not worked.
- It can be completed in a relatively short period of time.
- It can be provided in a variety of formats, including groups, self-help books, and apps.
- It teaches useful and practical strategies that can be used in daily life, even after treatment has ended.

Disadvantages of CBT:
- You must commit to the process to get the most out of it. A therapist can help guide you, but they'll need your cooperation.
- It can take up a good part of your time.
- It may not be appropriate for people who have more complex mental health needs or learning difficulties.
- It involves confronting your emotions and anxieties, so you may experience initial periods of anxiety or emotional discomfort.
- It focuses on the ability to change your thoughts, feelings, and behaviours. CBT does not address any external circumstances that may affect your health and well-being.[56]

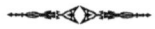

---

[56] https://www.nhs.uk/conditions/cognitive-behavioural-therapy-cbt/

Living Foods – The Essence of Life

"A healthy exterior starts from within."

~Robert Urich.

"The food you eat can be the safest and most powerful form of medicine or the slowest poison."

~Ann Wigmore.

You become what you eat

"You are what you eat, so don't be fast, cheap, easy, or fake." ~Anonymous.

The proverbial phrase "you are what you eat" means that you need to eat good food to be fit and healthy. This is literally true, because the structure and function of every cell in your body depends on the nutrients your food contains. You are constantly repairing and rebuilding your body. All the cells in your body have a fixed lifespan. Your body is busy creating new cells to replace those that have died. The health of these new cells depends on the quality of your diet. A nutritious and healthy diet can help you build healthy cells.[57]

Crash diets and their downfall

"Any food that requires chemical enhancement should not be considered food at all."

~ John H. Tobe.

---

[57] https://cynthiasass.com/sass-yourself/sass-yourself-blog/item/116-why-you-really-are-what-you-eat.html

Crash diets may offer an easy way to lose weight, but they are often inadequate, unsustainable, or unsafe. It is advisable to consult your doctor before trying any of these diets.

Some of the worst crash diets in history are:
- The clay diet.
- The air diet.
- The tapeworm's diet.
- The cookie diet.
- The Fletcher diet or *fletcherism*.
- The Sleeping Beauty Diet.
- The cotton ball diet.[58]

Characteristics of crash diets

- They have rigid and irrational rules. For example, they eat predominantly one type of food, such as grapefruit, meat, or cabbage soup.
- They require the elimination of entire food groups, such as carbohydrates or fats.
- They promise rapid weight loss, of one kilo per week or more.
- They severely restrict calorie consumption.
- They are often endorsed by celebrities.

Jumping from one crash diet to another can result in a rebound effect or yo-yo dieting. It's much more effective and healthy to make small, sustainable changes that last a lifetime.[59]

Meat, vegetarian or vegan

"Pay the farmer or pay the hospital."

---

[58] https://www.freshnlean.com/7-worst-fad-diets-history/
[59] https://mayoclinichealthsystem.org/hometown-health/speaking-of-health/dont-fall-for-a-fad-diet

~Birke Baehr.

Most people in Spain eat meat, but this number appears to be declining. Although vegetarians and vegans only make up a small percentage of the population, a significant number of people in a recent survey described their diet as "something other than non-vegetarian, vegan, and lacto-ovo vegetarian." Flexitarian diets (flexible vegetarian or semi-vegetarian) are becoming more popular.

People become vegetarians for many reasons, including health concerns, religious beliefs, the use of antibiotics and hormones in livestock, animal welfare concerns, or avoiding the overuse of environmental resources. Some people cannot afford to eat meat. Likewise, becoming vegetarian has become easier thanks to the availability of more vegetarian restaurant options, fresh vegetables, and the influence of Asian cultures with largely plant-based diets.

Meat is a good source of protein, B vitamins, and minerals such as iron, selenium, and zinc. However, meat is high in saturated fat. Furthermore, consumption of red and processed meats is linked to an increased risk of colon cancer. The general recommendation is to eat less than 500 grams of cooked meat per week and choose lean meats.

Vegetarian and vegan diets consist primarily of fruits, vegetables, whole grains, beans, legumes, lentils, nuts, and seeds. They contain very little saturated fat and are rich in dietary fibre. This may be why vegetarian and vegan diets are associated with a lower risk of obesity, high blood pressure, type 2 diabetes, heart disease, and cancer. According to the American Dietetic Association, "Appropriately planned vegetarian diets, including those that are totally vegetarian or vegan, are healthful, nutritionally adequate, and may provide health benefits in the prevention and treatment of certain diseases."

It's unclear whether these health benefits are due to any particular element of the diet or to all its components combined. Or whether it's because vegetarians and vegans are more health-conscious and make healthier lifestyle choices, such as being more active and avoiding smoking and excessive alcohol consumption. However, eating more fruits and vegetables likely provides significant health benefits.

Health risks of being vegetarian or vegan

The following deficiencies may be more common for vegans than for vegetarians:

Protein: Vegans can get their protein needs from many plant sources, including beans, lentils, chickpeas, peas, seeds, nuts, soy products, and whole grains.

Vitamin B12: Vitamin B12 is found only in animal products. Most vegetarians get their vitamin B12 from dairy products and eggs. Vegans should consume foods fortified with vitamin B12 or take a vitamin B12 supplement to avoid deficiencies that can cause pernicious anaemia and neurological problems.

Iron: The iron in meat is more easily absorbed than the iron found in plant foods, known as non-heme iron. However, it can be inhibited by phytic acid in whole grains, beans, lentils, seeds, and nuts.

Zinc: Vegetarians in Western countries do not appear to be deficient in zinc, although phytic acid in whole grains, seeds, beans, and legumes also reduces zinc absorption.

Omega-3 fatty acids: Omega-3 fatty acids may reduce inflammation, blood triglycerides, and even the risk of dementia. Diets that don't include fish or eggs are low in eicosapentaenoic acid (EPA) and docosahexaenoic acid (DHA). Plant foods typically contain only alpha linoleic acid (ALA). Our bodies can convert ALA from plant foods into EPA and DHA, but not very efficiently. Good sources of ALA include Brussels sprouts, flaxseed, chia seeds, hemp seeds, walnuts, canola oil, and soybeans. Vegans can also get their DHA from seaweed and algal oil supplements.

Balanced vegan or vegetarian diets can be a healthy choice. People choose to adopt a meat-free diet for a variety of reasons. However, eliminating meat completely may not be necessary for health reasons. A plant-based diet includes any diet that emphasises fruits, vegetables, plant proteins, and whole grains. For example, the Mediterranean diet includes many fruits and vegetables, beans, nuts, grains, and unsaturated fats (such as olive oil), but also includes fish and small amounts of dairy and meat products.

Changing our current diet to the pattern presented in this eating guide would result in an estimated 32% reduction in our carbon footprint, improving our health and helping to conserve the environment.[60]

Raw/processed

"If it came from a plant, eat it; if it was made in a plant, don't."
~Michael Pollan.

We are the only animals that process our food. Processed foods are those that are no longer in their natural state because they have been cooked or combined with other edible ingredients. For example, raw peanuts are in their natural state. However, roasted peanuts are no longer in their natural state because they have been cooked.[61]

A raw food diet consists mostly of raw plant foods, such as uncooked fruits and vegetables, nuts, seeds, fermented foods, and sprouted grains. It consists of at least 70% raw foods, almost always unheated, uncooked, and unprocessed.

Benefits of a raw food diet:
- Cooking foods deactivates the enzymes they contain. However, there is no evidence that enzymes contained in foods contribute to improved health.
- Some nutrients, particularly water-soluble vitamins, are lost during the cooking process.
- Raw fruits and vegetables may contain more nutrients, such as vitamins C and B.

Disadvantages of a raw food diet:
- Cooked foods are easier to chew and digest than raw foods.
- Cooking your vegetables can make some antioxidants more available to your body than they are in raw foods.

---

60 https://www.nutrition.org.uk/bnf-blogs/meatfree.html
61 http://www.bioedonline.org/lessons-and-more/lessons-by-topic/ecology/resources-and-the-environment/raw-vs-processed-food/

- Cooking food thoroughly kills bacteria that can cause some food-borne illnesses. This is especially true for meat, eggs, and dairy products.

Neither completely raw nor completely cooked diets can be justified by science. That's because fruits and vegetables, both raw and cooked, have several health benefits, including a lower risk of chronic diseases.[62]

Some foods are more nutritious when eaten raw, while others are more nutritious after being cooked.

- Foods that are healthier raw: broccoli, cabbage, garlic, onions.
- Foods that are healthier when cooked: asparagus, carrots, legumes, mushrooms, potatoes, spinach, tomatoes, meat, fish, and poultry.

Eat a combination of cooked and raw foods to maximise your health benefits. However, you don't need to follow a completely raw diet to maintain good health.[63]

Choose your foods better

"Let food be thy medicine and medicine be thy food." ~ Hippocrates.

Make your health a priority and take the time to take care of yourself.

1. Get nutrition information based on your age, gender, height, weight, and physical activity level.
2. Enjoy your food, but eat less. Use a smaller plate at meals to help you control the amount of food and calories you consume. Eat slowly and mindfully.
3. Make your plate half fruit and half vegetables. Choose red, orange, and green vegetables, such as tomatoes, potatoes, and broccoli, along with other greens. Eat fruit for dessert.
4. Drink water throughout the day to help maintain a healthy weight. Avoid carbonated drinks and alcohol.

---

62 http://cebp.aacrjournals.org/content/13/9/1422
63 https://www.healthline.com/nutrition/raw-food-vs-cooked-food

5. Choose whole grains, such as rice, pasta, and whole-wheat bread, more often. Foods high in fibre provide key nutrients and also keep you feeling full.
6. Use nutrition labels to discover the contents of different foods so you can make healthier choices.
7. Avoid or minimise foods high in saturated fat and added sugar. Limit processed meats, cakes, muffins, sweets, and ice cream.
8. Eat at home more often so you can control what you're eating. If you eat out, choose healthier options, such as baked chicken instead of fried.[64]

Balanced Diet - Is the Pyramid Still Applicable?

"You don't have to eat less; you just have to eat right."

~Anonymous.

The well-known food pyramid, introduced in 1991, was supposed to be our nutritional guide. However, many people found it confusing and didn't help us plan a healthy diet, one meal at a time. Most importantly, nutrition should be tailored to each individual because everyone is unique.

So, in May 2011, the U.S. Department of Agriculture finally scrapped the pyramid concept and replaced it with a plate. Its MyPyramid website was also revamped and redirected to a new website: www.ChooseMyPlate.gov.

While the basic nutritional guidelines for Americans remain the same, the old pyramid and the U.S. Department of Agriculture plate have several significant differences:

The food pyramid was dominated by grains, which filled the largest space at the bottom of the pyramid. This version of the plate reserves only one quadrant for grains (mostly whole grains) and allocates half of the plate to fruits and vegetables, more than any other food group. This is a huge improvement, as most of us don't eat enough fruits and vegetables.

---

[64] https://www.choosemyplate.gov/ten-tips-make-better-food-choices

Fats, oils, and sugars appeared in small amounts on the old pyramid, with the message that these foods should be consumed rarely or in small amounts. These foods do not appear anywhere on the plate, even though fat is essential for optimal health. However, ChooseMyPlate.gov offers in-depth information on fats, oils, and added sugars .

The Food Guide Pyramid told us how many portions of each food to consume each day. The plate doesn't list the portions to consume from any food group. The lack of portions makes the plate easier to implement and understand than the pyramid. Additionally, the ChooseMyPlate.gov website allows you to enter your personal information and obtain a personalised eating plan.

The pyramid only presented food groups, but the plate adds protein as one of the elements. Protein is a nutrient found in various foods, but it is not a food group. It seems out of place with fruits (food), vegetables (food), whole grains (food), and milk (food). Protein seems to be a simplification of the food group that includes meats, beans, nuts, and legumes. The U.S. Department of Agriculture says the term "protein" means a variety of sources, such as meat, eggs, dairy, nuts, seeds, beans, soy, etc.

The plate as an icon is easier to understand than the pyramid. Once you've seen it, it's easy to remember the message it conveys, as well as which food groups it includes. You can hang the *Choose My Plate symbol* on your kitchen wall as a reference guide. The goal is to match your dinner to all four quadrants of the plate for a balanced and nutritious meal.[65]

Ketogenic diet

"Healthy eating is a way of life, so it's important to establish routines that are simple, realistic, and ultimately liveable."

~ Horacio

A ketogenic or keto diet causes the body to release ketones into the blood.

Blood sugar, which comes from carbohydrates, is the body's primary source of energy. In the absence of blood sugar, we begin breaking down

---

[65] https://www.sparkpeople.com/resource/nutrition_articles.asp?id=425

stored fat into molecules called ketone bodies, using a process called ketosis. Once we're in ketosis, most cells will use ketone bodies to generate energy until we start consuming carbohydrates again.

The shift from using circulating glucose to breaking down stored fats as an energy source typically occurs over two to four days of eating fewer than 20 to 50 grams of carbohydrates per day.

Because it lacks carbohydrates, a ketogenic diet is rich in protein and fat. It typically includes plenty of meats, eggs, processed meats, sausages, cheeses, fish, nuts, butter, oils, seeds, and high-fibre vegetables. Because it's so restrictive, it's very difficult to follow long-term.

Carbohydrates typically make up at least 50% of a typical American diet. One of the biggest criticisms of this diet is that many people tend to eat too much low-quality protein and fat from processed foods, with too few fruits and vegetables. Patients with kidney failure should be cautious, as this diet could worsen their condition.

Is the ketogenic diet healthy?

Weight loss is the primary reason people often use the ketogenic diet. Previous research shows good evidence of rapid weight loss when patients adopt a ketogenic or very low-carb diet, compared to participants on a more traditional low-fat diet, or even a Mediterranean diet. However, this difference in weight loss appears to disappear over time.

A ketogenic diet has also been shown to improve blood sugar control for patients with type 2 diabetes in the short term. However, there is no research examining the diet's long-term effects on diabetes and high cholesterol.

Although a ketogenic diet can accelerate weight loss, it's difficult to follow and includes unhealthy foods, such as red meat and dairy. Its long-term effects are not well known, probably because it's so difficult to follow for so long! These crash diets, which lead to rapid weight loss and weight fluctuation, are associated with a high mortality rate. A balanced, plant-based diet, including colourful fruits and vegetables, whole grains, nuts, seeds, olive oil, fish, and lean meats, appears to be a better option than the keto diet.[66]

Pescatarian diet

"Every time you eat is an opportunity to nourish your body." ~Anonymous.

A pescatarian or pescavegetarian diet is a vegetarian diet that also includes fish as an additional source of protein. A pescatarian diet has many of the benefits of a plant-based diet, including reduced inflammation and a lower risk of diabetes and heart disease.

The pescatarian diet also helps to fill many of the nutritional gaps that can be present in a typical vegetarian diet, because fatty seafood contains beneficial vitamin D and omega-3 fatty acids. Seafood also contains iron, calcium, and vitamin B12, which can be lacking in many vegetarian diets.

One of the biggest disadvantages of a pescatarian diet is that some types of fish can have high levels of mercury, a neurotoxin linked to muscle weakness, loss of peripheral vision, impaired fine motor skills, tremors, headaches, insomnia, and emotional changes. Smaller fish tend to have much lower mercury content than larger fish, making them safer to eat.

Combining information from the U.S. Food and Drug Administration and the Environmental Protection Agency, the National Resources Defence Council grouped fish into four categories based on their mercury content:

Lowest in mercury (consume at will): anchovies, herring, North Atlantic mackerel, pollock, sardines, shrimp, freshwater trout, squid, clams, crayfish, and catfish.

Moderate mercury content (eat six servings or less per month): carp, cod, sea bass, mahi-mahi, lobster, snapper, freshwater perch, and canned chunk striped or albacore tuna.

High in mercury (three servings or less per month): halibut, sea perch, Chilean sea bass, albacore or white tuna, and Spanish mackerel.

---

[66] https://www.health.harvard.edu/blog/ketogenic-diet-is-the-ultimate-low-carb-diet-good-for-you-2017072712089

Higher mercury content (avoid these fish): bluefish, grouper, king mackerel, swordfish, bigeye tuna, shark, and emperor fish.[67]

Other disadvantages of a pescatarian diet include ethical issues surrounding fish farming and wild harvesting practices, such as the use of antibiotics, overfishing, and bycatch.[68]

Paleo diet

"Health is a relationship between you and your body."

~ Terri Guillemets.

The paleo diet is based on foods similar to those likely eaten during the Palaeolithic era, which roughly corresponds to a period between 2.5 million and 10,000 years ago. Other names for the paleo diet include the Palaeolithic diet, the Stone Age diet, the hunter-gatherer diet, and the caveman diet. The paleo diet includes foods that could be obtained through hunting and gathering in the past, such as lean meats, fish, fruits, vegetables, nuts, and seeds. A paleo diet limits foods such as dairy products, legumes, and whole grains, which became common when agriculture emerged around 10,000 years ago.

The goal of a paleo diet is to return to a way of eating that more closely resembles what primitive humans ate. This diet is said to help with weight loss and maintenance of a healthy weight.

Paleo diets follow these general guidelines:

Eat fruits, vegetables, nuts, seeds, lean meats (especially from grass-fed animals or wild birds), fish, and fruit and seed oils, such as olive or walnut oil.

Avoid whole grains, such as wheat, oats, and barley; legumes, such as beans, lentils, peanuts, and peas; dairy products; sugar, salt, potatoes, and highly processed foods in general.

---

67 https://www.nrdc.org/stories/smart-seafood-buying-guide
68 https://www.livestrong.com/article/399500-the-disadvantages-of-a-pescetarian-diet/

This diet also recommends drinking only water and staying physically active every day.

Several randomised clinical trials have compared the paleo diet to other diets, such as the Mediterranean diet. A paleo diet may provide benefits such as:

- Greater weight loss.
- Improvement in glucose tolerance.
- Better blood pressure control.
- Decrease in triglycerides.
- Better appetite management.

However, longer studies are needed to understand the long-term health benefits of the paleo diet.

Dietary concerns

The paleo diet is rich in vegetables, fruits, and nuts. However, it excludes whole grains and legumes, which are good sources of fibre, vitamins, and other nutrients. These foods are cheaper and more accessible than foods like wild birds, grass-fed animals, and nuts. Therefore, a paleo diet may be too expensive for some people.

You could achieve greater health benefits than the paleo diet by adopting a balanced, healthy diet that includes whole grains and legumes.[69]

Stool as an indicator of health

"If you can't pronounce it, don't eat it."

~ Michael Pollan.

Stool is primarily undigested food, proteins, bacteria, salts, and other substances produced and released by the intestines. Healthy stool varies widely.[70]

---

[69] https://www.mayoclinic.org/healthy-lifestyle/nutrition-and-healthy-eating/in-depth/paleo-diet/art-20111182
[70] https://www.healthline.com/health/digestive-health/types-of-poop

The Bristol Stool Scale is an indicator of different stool types. It is divided into seven categories, based on a study of 2,000 people.

Guy	Appearance	Indica
Type 1	Small, hard, separate lumps that look like nuts and are difficult to swallow.	These small lumps indicate that you're constipated. This shouldn't happen often.
Type 2	Shaped like a log, but bulging.	This is another sign of constipation that, again, shouldn't happen often.
Type 3	Shaped like a log with some cracks on the surface.	This is the gold standard for stool, especially if it is somewhat soft and easy to pass.
Type 4	Smooth and snake-like.	Doctors also consider this type of stool as something normal that should happen every one to three days.
Type 5	These are small, like the first ones, but soft and easy to pass. The amorphous masses also have defined edges.	This type of stool indicates that you are lacking fibre and should find ways to add it to your diet through eating grains or vegetables.
Type 6	Spongy and loose, with irregular edges.	This overly soft consistency could be a sign of mild diarrhoea. Try drinking more water and fruit juice to help improve this condition.
Type 7	Completely watery with no solid pieces.	In other words, you have diarrhoea. This means your stool passed through your intestines too quickly and didn't turn into healthy stool.

Stool colour: Stool comes in a variety of colours. All shades of brown, and even green, are considered normal. The colour of stool is influenced by what you eat, as well as the amount of bile it contains (bile is a yellow-green fluid that digests fats). Seek immediate medical attention if your stool is bright red or black, as this could indicate the presence of blood.

Excrement Quality	What it can mean	Possible dietary causes
Green	Food may be passing through the large intestine too quickly, as in diarrhoea. As a result, the bile doesn't have time to fully break down.	Green leafy vegetables; green food colouring, such as that found in flavoured drink mixes or ice cream; iron supplements.
Light, white or clay-coloured	Absence of bile in the stool. This may indicate a bile duct obstruction.	Certain medications, such as high doses of bismuth subsalicylate (Kaopectate, Pepto-Bismol) and other antidiarrheal medications.
Yellow, greasy, bad smelling	Excess fat in the stool, such as that caused by a malabsorption disorder, such as celiac disease.	Sometimes gluten, a protein like that found in bread and cereals, can cause a problem. Get evaluated by a doctor.
Black	Bleeding in the upper intestinal tract, such as the stomach.	Iron supplements, bismuth subsalicylate (Kaopectate, Pepto-Bismol), Licorice.
Bright red	Bleeding from the lower intestinal tract, such as the large intestine or rectum, often due to hemorrhoids.	Red food colouring, beets, cranberries, tomato juice or soup, gelatin, or red drink mixes.

Best Recommendations

"Moderation. Small portions. Try a little bit of everything. These are the secrets to happiness and good health."

~ Julia Child.

Most diets, including raw food, vegan, paleo, and keto, are not sustainable for long periods of time due to individual lifestyles, food preferences, lack of support, etc.

Your long-term health results depend on your behaviour, not your diet. To maintain a healthy body and weight, you must develop consistent and sustainable daily habits. For example, instead of consuming 800 calories one day and 3,000 calories the next, aim to consume just a little more than the amount you can maintain and gradually reduce it over time, if necessary. Aim for progress in small amounts (*kaizen*).

Other healthy strategies you can adopt while enjoying the foods you love:

- Eat slowly and consciously.
- Eat until you are 80% full.
- Eat less processed foods.
- Eat more fibre and protein.
- Get high-quality sleep more often.
- Move throughout the day and minimise sedentary lifestyle.
- Exercise regularly to improve your strength, endurance, flexibility, and balance.
- Take action to reduce stress and build resilience (meditation).
- Spend quality time with family and friends.[71]

---

[71] https://www.precisionnutrition.com/calories-in-calories-out

Time - The enigma of life

"Healing is an art. It takes time. It takes practice. It takes love."
~Maza Dohta.

"Protecting and maintaining your body's innate ability to be healthy and heal depends on you: on making the right choices about how to live." ~Andrew Weil.

Healing takes time

Good health requires time and commitment. Your symptoms didn't develop overnight. They're typically a gradual but progressive accumulation of toxicity and physical changes.

However, this is the age of instant gratification. Most of us tend to be impatient and want instant relief. Unfortunately, instant relief is not healing. Instant relief masks our symptoms without restoring the body to its natural, healthy state.

For example, most medications provide instant relief by masking our symptoms. So, you have to keep taking them to continue receiving relief. But when we discontinue the medication, the symptoms return almost immediately. Ideally, the medication should correct the problem so we can stop taking it after a reasonable period. Usually, this isn't the case.

For example, have you ever known someone whose diabetes medications healed so much that they could stop taking them? What about high blood pressure? Migraines? Heart disease? We're typically forced to take these medications for life because they can control these disorders, but not reverse or cure them.

On the other hand, a nutrition and lifestyle programme addresses the true causes of your illness. If you stick with the programme for the prescribed time, you'll improve and regain your health.

True healing takes time. It can take several months to fully recover from a chronic health problem. It might even take several years to fully overcome a degenerative condition.

How long is a reasonable time to heal?

The time it takes to heal depends on many factors, such as the nature of your disorder, your immunity, the severity and duration of the illness, etc. With acute illnesses, improvement is usually faster. Chronic illnesses take longer to improve. Degenerative diseases can take even longer, especially if they involve organs, bones, and joints.

Getting better means you should feel better. The true test of any therapy is how it affects your body and mind. Do you feel more energetic? Is your sense of well-being improving? Do you feel more alive and healthy? You need to learn to listen to your own body and trust what it's telling you.

When the cause of your illness is eliminated, you will notice that your symptoms diminish and your energy levels increase. Conversely, if your body cannot eliminate the cause of your illness, it will overpower your body's defence mechanisms. This leads to stagnation, decreased energy levels, and the progressive weakening of your organic systems.

There are two reasons why healing fails:
- Your body's immunity was too weak to resist and overcome the irritant. That's why the foundation of medicine is restoring immunity and health.
- Your immune response is suppressed by painkillers and other medications. Symptoms like fever, runny nose, sneezing, diarrhoea, cough, etc. are ways of eliminating irritants. Instant symptom relief with medications interferes with these body's natural responses. When you take these medications, your body isn't truly healed.

The problem hides and develops into a chronic or degenerative disease.[72]

There are a vast number of challenges our bodies can face, each responding differently, and each person's response is unique. What we do know is that true healing and correction isn't instantaneous (and, if it were, it would be unsustainable). Time is the KEY to achieving true change. Small, targeted, and sustained changes lead to the biggest and most sustainable change. Be patient with your body; it has certainly been patient with you.

Patients often say their age is the reason they feel and look the way they do, but is this necessarily true? Does age affect healing? Is age associated with longer healing times? Let's take a look.

Why does the body age and how does it age?

Aging is a complex process that affects different people, and even different organs, in different ways. No single process can explain all the changes that occur with aging. This is due to the interaction of many influences throughout life, including heredity, environment, diet, exercise, past illnesses, genes, lifestyle, and many other factors.

The cause and mechanism of aging are unclear. It could be a predetermined process, controlled by genes; or it could be due to long-term damage caused by ultraviolet light or metabolic byproducts, such as free radicals.

Each person ages differently. Although some changes always occur with aging, they do so at different rates and extents . Some systems begin aging as early as age 30. Other aging processes aren't common until much later in life. There's no way to predict exactly how you'll age.[73]

---

[72] https://www.webnat.com/articles/Healing.asp
[73] https://medlineplus.gov/ency/article/004012.htm

Is degeneration associated with age?

Our bodies change with age due to changes in individual cells and organs. These changes result in changes in function and appearance. Some age-related functional changes include:

Mental function

Difficulty learning new material: The number of nerve cell receptors may decrease. Therefore, the brain doesn't send or process impulses as well or as quickly.

Physical activity

Instability or loss of balance: The structures of the inner ear that help maintain balance stiffen and deteriorate slightly. The part of the brain that controls balance (cerebellum) may degenerate.

Dizziness or lightheadedness upon standing: The heart doesn't send enough blood to the head because it's less able to respond to changes in position. Veins and arteries don't constrict enough to maintain normal blood pressure when the person stands.

Loss of muscle strength: The number and size of muscle fibres decreases. The body produces less growth hormone (and less testosterone in men).

Difficulty moving and decreased flexibility: Less synovial fluid is produced. Muscle tissue is lost, decreasing strength and causing muscles to stiffen.

Difficulty performing vigorous exercise: The heart cannot handle the demand for more blood and the lungs cannot handle the demand for oxygen during exercise.

The senses

Need for reading glasses: The lens of the eye hardens, making it more difficult to focus on close objects.

Difficulty seeing in dim light: The retina of the eye becomes less sensitive to light and the lens loses transparency.

Difficulty adjusting to changes in light levels: Pupils react more slowly to changes in light.

Dry eyes: The number of cells that produce fluid to lubricate the eyes decreases. The tear glands secrete fewer tears.

Hearing loss: Age-related hearing loss (presbycusis) develops.

Loss of taste: Taste buds become less sensitive.

Dry mouth: Less saliva is produced.

Eating disorders

Difficulty swallowing: The mouth is dry. People may not chew food enough because of tooth loss or poorly fitting dentures.

Lack of interest in food: The senses of taste and smell diminish, making food less appetising.

Skin and hair

Wrinkles: The layer of fat under the skin decreases.

Dry skin: The glands in the skin produce less oil.

Lesions: The arteries and veins of the skin become more fragile.

Decreased sensation: The number of nerve endings in the skin decreases.

Gray or white hair: Hair follicles produce less pigment (melanin).

Hair thinning or loss: Some hair follicles stop producing new hair.

Sexual function

Vaginal dryness: Less oestrogen is produced.

Erections that don't last as long, are less rigid, or take longer to develop: Less testosterone is produced. Blood flow to the penis is reduced.[74]

However, there's no need to feel overly depressed or anxious. Most of the significant health issues associated with aging can be minimised with a healthy lifestyle and a positive attitude. As Mark Twain said, "Age is a

---

[74] https://www.merckmanuals.com/home/older-people%E2%80%99s-health-issues/the-aging-body/changes-in-the-body-with-aging

matter of mind over body. If you don't mind it, it doesn't matter." He also said, "Wrinkles should be only a marker of where smiles once were."

Age-related loss of flexibility

In older adults, ages 55 to 85, age-related flexibility loss appears to be so minimal that normal loss of joint range of motion does not appear to affect daily functions or cause disability.[75]

Many age-related changes, including decreased flexibility, are caused by disuse and a sedentary lifestyle. Men are more likely to experience decreased flexibility than women.

Exercise and yoga can reverse many age-related changes, including the loss of flexibility. However, exercise should be approached with caution, with long warm-ups and stretches, and adequate recovery to prevent injury, especially if you have been sedentary. It's best to seek professional guidance.[76]

Time, movement, hydration, balanced nutrition, and a positive mental attitude are all vital elements in healing, and all must be addressed when actively working toward health. Be patient and coordinate your efforts; it's really that simple.

---

[75] https://www.hindawi.com/journals/jar/2013/743843/
[76] https://www.naturalathleteclinic.com/blogs/natural-athlete-solutions/preventing-age-related-declines-in-flexibility

Water – The elixir of life

"You're 87% water; the other 13% keeps you from drowning."
~PE Morris.

"Drinking water is like washing yourself internally. Water will cleanse your system, replenish it, reduce your caloric load, and improve the function of all your tissues."
~Kevin R. Stone

Good hydration is vital for good health.

Water makes up about two-thirds of your body and approximately 73% of your brain. [77]Every organ in your body needs water to function properly. You need water to maintain your body temperature, eliminate waste, lubricate your joints, and maintain good overall health. [78]Good hydration has been shown to reduce the risk of many health conditions, including constipation, hypertension, kidney stones, urinary tract infections, and exercise-induced asthma.[79]

How much water do you need?

Water is essential for maintaining normal physical and cognitive functions, and for normal thermoregulation. [80]According to the European

---

[77] Mitchell HH et al. (1945) «The chemical composition of the adult human body and its bearing on the biochemistry of growth». *Journal of Biological Chemistry* 158(3): 625-37
[78] https://www.ncbi.nlm.nih.gov/pubmed/19724292
[79] https://www.ncbi.nlm.nih.gov/pubmed/16028566
[80] EFSA (2011) «Scientific Opinion on the substantiation of health claims related to water and maintenance of normal physical and cognitive functions (ID 1102, 1209, 1294, 1331), maintenance of normal thermoregulation (ID 1208) and

Food Safety Authority's scientific estimate of water consumption, men should consume a total of 2.5 litres of water per day, while women should consume a total of 2 litres of water per day. Ideally, 70–80% of this should consist of beverages and 20–30% of food.[81]

Average water intake = 2.5 litres	Average water consumption = 2.5 litres
Water in liquids: 1.5 litres	Urine: 1.6 litres
Food water: 0.7 litres	Sweat: 0.45 litres
Metabolic water: 0.3 litres	Breathing: 0.35 litres
	Feces: 0.2 litres
Total: 2.5 litres	**Total: 2.5 litres**

Water balance in sedentary adults living in temperate climates[82]

Typically, food contributes 20–30% of total dietary fluid intake, while beverages account for 70–80%. This ratio is not fixed and depends on the type of beverage and food choice. Foods have a wide range of water contents (from less than 40% to more than 80%).

Your water intake needs change throughout the day. Ideally, your water intake should equal your 24-hour water needs.[83]

If water intake is lower than required, we become dehydrated. This is more likely to occur in dry conditions, especially if we have limited access to water and lose more water than normal through exercise, sweat, diarrhoea, or vomiting.

Mild dehydration can occur when we lose 1-2 percent of our body weight. Some symptoms of mild to moderate dehydration include thirst,

---

basic requirement of all living things» (ID 1207) pursuant to Article 13(1) of Regulation (EC) No 1924/2006. *EFSA Journal* 9(4):2075
[81] EFSA (2010) «Scientific Opinion on Dietary Reference Values for water». *EFSA Journal* 8(3):1459
[82] https://www.ncbi.nlm.nih.gov/pubmed/19724292
[83] https://www.ncbi.nlm.nih.gov/pmc/articles/PMC4207053/

dark-coloured urine, decreased urination, fatigue, dizziness, constipation, and confusion.[84]

Different forms of liquids

Water: Science has proven the truth of this ancient Slovak proverb: "Pure water is the first and greatest medicine." Water has zero calories and is the best way to quench thirst. Drink plain water. You don't need to drink bottled water. Tap water is good enough. However, you may need to filter it before drinking it. To make the water more refreshing, add a lemon or lime wheel.

Tea and coffee: You should limit your daily caffeine intake to about 400 mg, which is equivalent to 750 ml of black coffee (3 cups) or 1 litre of black tea per day (4 cups). If you're pregnant, limit your caffeine intake to 500 ml of coffee (2 cups) or 750 ml of tea (3 cups). Drink herbal tea or decaffeinated coffee if you want to consume more than the recommended amount of caffeinated beverages. Avoid *gourmet coffees and teas*, as they contain more sugar.

Fruit and vegetable juices: Limit your consumption of fruit juices, as they are high in calories and low in fibre. Instead, eat fruit. Make sure to choose 100% real fruit juices. Avoid fruit drinks or cocktails, as these contain added sugars and few nutrients.

Broths and Soups: Broths and broth-based soups are a good source of fluids. However, most canned soups and broths have too much added salt. Choose low-sodium soups or make your own.

Carbonated drinks: Avoid these drinks because they are high in calories, sugars, and chemicals. Some carbonated drinks, such as colas, may also contain caffeine. Diet carbonated drinks have no calories or sugar, but they may contain caffeine, sweeteners, and other chemicals.

Sports drinks: Commercial sports drinks are generally not necessary to maintain hydration during exercise. Many of them contain unhealthy

---

[84] https://www.mayoclinic.org/diseases-conditions/dehydration/symptoms-causes/syc-20354086

ingredients. Water and a healthy diet can replace the water and minerals lost during exercise.[85]

Alcohol: Minimise alcoholic beverages. The immediate effects of cutting back on alcohol include feeling better in the morning, being less tired throughout the day, improving skin appearance, feeling more energetic, and better weight management. Long-term benefits include improvements in mood, sleep, judgment, memory, immunity, behaviour, and overall health.[86] The next time you're tempted to drink alcohol with friends, remember this wise Chinese proverb: "With true friends… even water drunk together is sweet enough."

Dehydration

A survey conducted by the Royal National Lifeboat Institution showed that 89% of the population is not drinking enough water to maintain healthy hydration levels. Men are much less hydrated than women: 20% of men don't drink any water during the day, compared to 13% of women. Older people are less hydrated: 25% of people over 55 reported not drinking water during the day, compared to 7% of people aged 25-34.[87]

Top tips for healthy hydration

1. Drink water. It's the best way to hydrate and has no calories, sugars, or artificial chemicals. Heed these words from Thoreau: "Water is the only drink of a wise man."
2. Choose foods high in water content, such as soups, stews, vegetables, and fruits, to increase your total daily water intake.
3. Drink water regularly throughout the day because hydration levels fluctuate throughout the day.
4. Drink more water when you exercise or spend time in hot, dry environments.

---

[85] https://www.dietitians.ca/getattachment/becace49-3bad-4754-ac94-f31c3f04fed0/FACTSHEET-Guidelines-for-staying-hydrated.pdf.aspx
[86] https://www.nhs.uk/live-well/alcohol-support/tips-on-cutting-down-alcohol/
[87] https://www.naturalhydrationcouncil.org.uk/press/how-hydrated-is-britain/

5. Make sure you carry water with you, especially when travelling. Keep your water close to you when you're at work, school, or playing.
6. Make sure you're drinking pure water. Use a filter if necessary.
7. Avoid or minimise unhealthy beverages, such as soda, caffeinated beverages, and alcohol.[88]

Final tip – listen to your body

Check your thirst: If you're thirsty or have a dry mouth, you may not be drinking enough water. Remember, when you're thirsty, you're already somewhat dehydrated. Try to drink fluids often throughout the day.

Check your urine: If your urine is dark yellow and has a strong odour, you may not be getting enough fluids. Light yellow or colourless urine usually indicates that you're getting enough fluids. The amount of urine you produce can also be a sign of your hydration status. If you don't urinate much throughout the day and your urine is dark in colour, you need more fluids.

Check your mood: If you feel tired and can't concentrate or have headaches, these could be signs that you're dehydrated.[89]

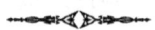

---

[88] Dr. Emma Derbyshire PhD, National Hydration Council, *The Essential Guide to Hydration*

[89] https://www.unlockfood.ca/en/Articles/Water/Facts-on-Fluids-How-to-Stay-Hydrated.aspx

Farewell words

"Health is the new wealth. We will continue to define success by how nice our house is or the area we live in. But going forward, health will increasingly be synonymous with social status. Health will be a currency in itself. You can't necessarily buy health, but you will know how to get it, and you can get it every day of your life."

~ Henry Loubet, *CEO,* Bohemia Health.

"Never doubt that a small group of thoughtful, committed citizens can change the world; in fact, it's the only thing in history that has ever done so."

~Margaret Mead.

Congratulations on finishing the book! Whether you read every page or just the chapters that interested you, you've already taken the first step. You're great!

Nine out of ten people who buy books don't finish them. This is why Groucho Marx said, "From the moment I held your book in my hands until I put it down, I was convulsing with laughter. Someday I'll read it."

You're part of the small minority of people who have decided to take charge of their health and seek information and help. That's the right first step.

As I've already explained, the vital principles that will help you achieve your health goals are:

- Chiropractic and health.
- Exercise.
- The change of attitude.
- Food.

- The weather.

- Hydration.

The most important lesson from this book is that you must take responsibility for your own health, nourishing your body and mind. And this starts with making the right choices.

A journey of a thousand miles begins with the first step. Choose a small step you can take right now. Do a single plank or squat. Or drink a glass of water. Or spend more quality time with your family. Whatever it is, stop reading and do it right now.

A final warning: each of us is different and has different health issues, determined by our age, gender, genes, environment, emotions, and past illnesses. Please consult your doctor before making any important decisions that could affect your health.

I hope this book has been helpful. If you have any questions or comments, please contact us at www.thamechiropracticclinic.com or 01844 212100. We would love to hear from you.

All the best on your journey to a happy, healthy, and harmonious life!

"Eternal happiness isn't a fairy tale, it's a choice."

~Fawn Weaver.

About the Author

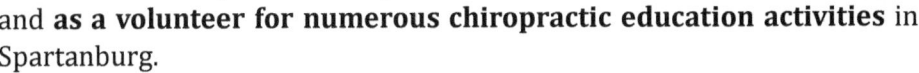

Arthur Tovar, D.C.

Arthur Tovar graduated as a Doctor in Chiropractic from Sherman College of Straight Chiropractic, (Spartanburg, S.C.) USA in 2005 with a magna *cum laude*.

He also served as vice-president and instructor of the Sacro-Occipital Technique Club for two years and **as a volunteer for numerous chiropractic education activities** in Spartanburg.

He holds certifications with National Board of Chiropractic Examiners in Part I, II, III, IV and Physiotherapy. He has been licensed in the State of Massachusetts where he first started practice in the USA. And holds a Bachelor of Science degree from Excelsior College in New York.

He holds certification in Webster Technique with the ICPA (International Chiropractic Paediatrics Association)

He is a member of SOTO USA and Soto Europe in SOT Technique (Sacro Occipital Technique)

He has helped teaching SOT Technique with SOTO Europe to Chiropractors.

He is a board certified Craniopath with SOTO USA.

He is a member of the ICPA.

He holds advanced certification in Applied Kinesiology with the ICAK in the UK

He is the author of numerous health articles, some published in national magazines, and videos on how to achieve a better quality of life naturally.

He has also published a case review in Facial palsy with the Asian Pacific Chiropractic Journal https://thamechiropracticclinic.com/wp-content/uploads/2020/12/Tovar-Facial-Palsy-SOT-RC-2019-1.3-PDF.pdf.

Since 2007, he has dedicated himself to improving the health and lives of people in the Oxfordshire area through chiropractic care.

You can find more information at www.thamechiropracticclinic.com

www.ingramcontent.com/pod-product-compliance
Lightning Source LLC
Chambersburg PA
CBHW060033040426
42333CB00042B/2412